KETOGENIC DIET

Understand Ketogenic Diets in Under an Hour

Christopher Smith

TABLE OF CONTENTS

INTRODUCTION:

For the vast majority of people the word "diet" brings to mind a condition where, for a few days or weeks, we eat less than what we usually do, in order to lose some extra weight. And then what happens? After this period is ended and we have achieved the required results, we get back to eating as usual. What is the result? We gain back the weight we lost and then some.

The only other reason that a person would go on a diet is because the doctor said so. There are plenty of medical conditions that can be remedied or assisted if the dietary habits of a person change. Usually these diets are chemical in nature and intended to take advantage of certain reactions that occur in the body.

Actually that's what all diets are looking for... the opportunity to take advantage of what is going on inside the body so that they can achieve their objective. While most of them succeed, their results are not permanent unless there is a radical change not only on the processes inside the body, but also in the way of thinking of each individual.

This is the premise of a ketogenic diet. You must force the body to abandon glucose as its main source of energy and switch to ketones. The relevant research shows that some organs of the body like the brain, the heart and the kidneys work better if their energy comes from ketones.

The discovery of this kind of diet is not new. It dates back all the way to the 1920s when an alternative was looked for to overcome the catatonia and muscle loss that were the most common side effects of the fasting of the era. The medical community needed to maintain the results without the side effects. What they came up with is the ketogenic diet which will be explored and discussed in this book.

Before proceeding any further it must be made abundantly clear that under no circumstances it is to be considered that the contents of this book intend to replace the advice and the guidance provided by a proper medical professional.

Quite the opposite, it is strongly recommended that you receive such advice before making the decision to proceed in the implementation of a ketogenic diet. There may be underlying medical conditions involved that could be prohibitive and should be attended to by other means.

Furthermore, as it will be pointed out herein, there will be issues that will require the supervision of such a professional throughout the implementation of a ketogenic diet.

Actually there have been a lot of questions posed as to the effectiveness of such a change in the dietary habits to people suffering from both types of diabetes. It is a matter of fact that the diet was and is conceived as a means of medical therapy and not as a simple diet and therefore such is the way it should be regarded.

While explaining the changes that must be implemented when someone decides to go on a ketogenic diet, it will be evident that these changes will be of a permanent nature. And that raises even more questions and issues which will find a response and an explanation in the following chapters.

This issue of permanent changes re-enforces the suggestion for proper medical guidance and supervision. Even if everything looks good in the beginning, there have been rare instances that conditions arose later on in the therapy that forced the abandonment of the diet.

No matter the reason behind going on a ketogenic diet, or any diet for that matter, there is always the issue that needs to base the results of the diet upon the decision. You need to make a definite and permanent decision to go on a diet and you need to make a similar decision to maintain the new lifestyle on a permanent basis. The contents of this book intend for your decision to be fully informed.

WHAT IS KETOSIS AND HOW IT WORKS

WHAT HAPPENS WHEN WE EAT?

We all know that the vast majority of our food intake in the contemporary western diets consists of carbohydrates. Eating carbohydrates forces the body to use glucose as the primary source of energy. If there is not enough glucose in the carbohydrates consumed, or if this consumption is significantly lowered, then, in order to procure the necessary glucose, the body will burn some fat.

This fat may have just been consumed as a "guacamole on the side" order, or taken out of the body's deposits of fat around the waist, which is the required process when we want to lose some weight. The interesting twist of nature here is that while the body can use glucose to produce fat, the opposite function has not been written in the body's computers, nor has any way been found by science to include such a function in the human cells artificially.

When fat is thrown into the boiler (to borrow from the image of an old steam engine and the process of shoveling coal into it), most of it is directly converted to what is known as ATP (scientifically called adenosine triphosphate). ATP gets the chemical energy and transfers it to the various cells during the metabolism phase.

The remaining part of fat is converted to ketone bodies. There seems to be a misconception here. The ketone bodies that are used in the ketogenic diet have nothing to do with the ketones which are pervasive in nature. In fact, there are only three molecules involved in this process: acetone, acetoacetic acid and beta-hydroxyboutyric acid.

The less glucose is available to be used for energy the more ketones are produced. To avoid any misunderstandings, ketones are produced at all times. The body turns to them for energy after the default, so to speak, quantity has been produced and there is no glucose for the additional amounts required.

WHAT IS KETOSIS?

The point of the exercise of a ketogenic diet is to force the body to abandon glucose and turn to ketones for its energy. The kidneys and the heart muscle use the default amount of ketones produced as they work better with them than glucose. All the other organs can adapt to ketones at least for the major part of energy they require.

When we reduce the consumption of carbohydrates, the enforcement described above takes place. The first indication that the body has turned into the process of burning the stored fat is the production of acetone which is detectable in the excretions of the body. This is called ketosis and it is not a dangerous process as many people may think.

This is the main reason that there must be medical supervision present. The levels of acetone must be closely monitored as if a certain level is exceeded it may mean that there is ketoacidosis occurring and this is a condition to be treated in a medical facility.

KETOACIDOSIS

People have been avoiding ketogenic diets because they think that they may be in danger. This actually happens in people suffering from diabetes, either of type I, which is a result of lack of insulin, or of type II which is insulin dependent.

Their ketone levels are higher to start with. A ketogenic diet may result in a production of more ketones than necessary which in turn may result in ketoacidosis. At least that's what the people who avoid it maintain. Recent research has actually shown that it is not the diet that is responsible for the higher levels of ketones but a rather complex set of circumstances that result from the condition itself. As we will explain in the next chapter, people suffering from diabetes will actually benefit from turning to a ketogenic diet.

A word of warning is in order at this point. If you decide to change your dietary habits as described herein, there will be a transitional period of about a week. This period is required for the body to adjust and while it lasts you may experience weariness, headaches, weakness, some mild irritability and light-headedness.

These are all expectable symptoms and should not make you worry. If they do worry you or if you need to overcome them, you can turn to performance enhancers which will mitigate these symptoms after receiving relevant advice and guidance by your physician.

The combination of foods described in this book is generic. Some adjustments may be required until the optimal results are reached. In the vast majority of cases, nutritional ketosis is reached between 2 and 4 weeks after the diet has commenced, however, this period may be longer depended on your own specific circumstances.

If you are an athlete and have decided to turn to such a diet, you may experience these symptoms for a longer period of time at lower intensity. For you, the complete adaptation of your body may take up as much as 12 weeks.

We have already discussed that the diet was initially researched as a medical treatment. Let's explore in the next chapter how it affects some conditions.

WHAT CONDITIONS ARE HELPED WITH KETOSIS

The original concept of the research for a ketogenic diet was to maintain the benefits of fasting without the side-effects of muscle loss and catatonia. After 70 years of going through the results of the tests, the evidence that such a diet is beneficial finds the optimal expression in the following conditions:

ACNE

Acne can be a result of insulin resistance which creates a host of favourable conditions for the hormonal side of acne. Insulin is directly linked to the existence of glucose. By eliminating glucose, this connection is reduced resulting to a reduction of the insulin resistance and therefore diminishing one of the underlying causes of acne.

BRAIN CANCER AND OTHER FORMS OF CANCER

Cancer cells require glutamine and glucose to survive. Without glucose they are actually deprived of their sustenance and they starve to death. Unfortunately in this case it is not the diet that presents any problems. It is the resistance of the patients to even consider changing their dietary habits which mounts up to a staggering 70% of the cases.

DIABETES

We have already mentioned a few things superficially. Let's take a deeper look on the exact effects of the diet to both types of diabetes, especially type 2. First of all the high levels of glucose in the blood are one of the primary causes of diabetes. Secondly almost all diabetics are overweight. A ketogenic diet will both reduce the blood levels of glucose and the weight which in turn will reduce the dependency on medication and its side effects.

It should be repeated at this point that the level of ketones in diabetics must be closely monitored to avoid the development of ketoacidosis.

EPILEPSY

In fact this is the first of the medical conditions that were examined in relation with a ketogenic diet. The results were so impressive that it is recommended in almost all cases of the appearance of the condition in children. The seizures are reduced by 50% and a percentage of 15 – 20% of the children can live a completely seizure free life. There are only two reasons that prohibit the implementation of this treatment: The existence of mitochondrial and metabolic disorders.

NEUROLOGICAL CONDITIONS

This is a bit trickier to explain in a few words. To put it as simply as possible, a ketogenic diet will enhance the levels of neuronal energy. This energy will make it possible to transfer neuro-protective agents that will provide protection against a number of types of cellular activity. By protecting the nerves the symptoms of conditions like Amyotrophic Lateral Sclerosis, brain trauma, Alzheimer's and narcolepsy are relieved. Furthermore, the activity related to these diseases is changed and the nerves become stronger and more resistant to their effects. Especially in brain conditions, a ketogenic diet will result in a reduction of the possibility of strokes.

P.O.S.

The scientific name is Polycystic Ovarian Syndrome and it affects women at their reproductive ages. It is directly related to insulin resistance and obesity much like diabetes and it has already been adequately mentioned how the elimination of glucose will both reduce the insulin resistance and the overweight, therefore, benefiting the syndrome.

RISK OF CARDIOVASCULAR DISEASES

The built up of arterial plaque is the main reason of increasing the risk of cardiovascular diseases. Controlling HDL and LDL and their ratio to triglycerides controls the build up of the plaque. As long as there is no more than the absolutely required level of glucose this build up is kept below risk levels.

The list could include other medical conditions that may benefit directly or indirectly from the elimination of glucose and the basing of the energy source to ketones. Let's take a deeper look on how this is achieved.

THE COMBINATION OF CARBOHYDRATES, FAT AND PROTEIN

If one was to break down the foods that we are eating, it would be very easy to see that they belong to three basic categories: Fat, proteins and carbohydrates. These three categories provide the values that the human body requires to work efficiently. Anything more than the values that the body can tolerate will result in the glucose been converted to fat with all the effects that we are well aware of.

A ketogenic diet is based on the optimal per case combination for consumption of these three categories. The premises for each category are the following:

Protein

Proteins are the building blocks of the body. They are the ones that counteract the muscle loss issue when fasting. Therefore, they need to be included in every form of diet. In this case they are not as necessary when the diet is at its first stages as later on. Their use is to maintain nutritional ketosis which necessitates supervision as overconsumption of protein may result in the diet losing its capacity to produce ketones.

Furthermore, for many people, it is a more natural process for their bodies to engage in gluconeogenesis (convert protein to glucose). Strict control of protein intake must be exercised at all times to avoid such an occurrence.

Carbohydrates

The carbohydrates (or carbs as most commonly referred to), in this instance act as regulators. Their percentage in the diet determines the levels of ketone production for the followed diet. The amount of permissible daily consumption is determined by the age, metabolism parameters and physical condition of the body in each specific case.

For normal values in the above parameter the consumption should be between 50 and 60 grams per day. Athletes and people in better shape could go up to 100 grams, but older people may have to reduce the quantity to as low as 30 grams. This is another reason that the supervision of a physician is required.

The amount of grams is determined after the deduction from the daily total intake of carbs, of the amount of the carbs consumed that corresponds to fibers and sugar alcohols. Fibers and sugar alcohols cannot be used to produce energy. Therefore the number of grams mentioned above corresponds to the actual amount of carbs that is effective, i.e. usable to produce energy.

If you consume a cup of raw broccoli, you get 4 grams of carbohydrates. Half of them come from fibers which cannot produce calories. Based on the above principle the effective amount in this case is 2 grams.

FAT

The part that matters the most as it is what will be converted to energy and the part that counteracts the effect of catatonia. Calculating the exact amount to be consumed per day is a subject of the percentages of carbs and protein, the daily activities of each individual which determine the number of calories required, the amount of stored fat in the body and the requirements on how much weight is to be lost in a certain amount of time.

The first positive thing to know about eating fat, is that people that are aware they are consuming it, tend not to overeat which reduces the chance of a greater intake than necessary. 60 to 80% of the calories required will come from fat. For the treatment of epilepsy this percentage can go up as high as 90%.

The important issue to consider is the kind of fat that must be included in the dietary habits. Fats belonging to the omega 6 family (polyunsaturated fats like sunflower and corn) are to be completely removed. They can be inflammatory and they do not serve their purpose in ketosis.

The easiest fats to be converted to ketones are those with high concentration of medium chain triglycerides and monounsaturated and saturated fats like olive oil, coconut oil, cheese, avocados and butter. For sunflower oil, any consumption should include only the high oleic form.

Again, there must be supervision especially if the fats consumed are saturated. Such consumption may affect the blood lipid profile. It is the profile that determines abnormalities in the triglycerides and cholesterol.

To begin the process of getting the body into ketosis the usual process is to consume no carbohydrates for the first couple of days while the ration of fat to protein mix in the meals should be 80 – 20 percent. Gradually the amount of fat must be reduced, the carbohydrates introduced into the diet and the protein increased until the ratios become about 5% carbs, 65% fat and 30% proteins. Most of the carbohydrates must come from fiber.

Now that the theory behind the concept is established, it is time to go into what really matters for those that wish to switch to a ketogenic diet which is the daily meals.

COMPLETE DAILY MENUS

The mere sound of the word "diet" predetermines the listener about a set of meals that will not taste as good as a nice juicy steak seasoned with salt, mustard, ketchup and pepper, or a burger covered with cheese and bacon. To paraphrase a known aphorism the road to a bad lifestyle is paved with tasty delicacies.

Some of the suggestions for a full set of daily meals may actually cover the second part of the aphorism but preclude the first one:

MENU SUGGESTION 1:

Breakfast: Pour 1/2 cup of boiling water into a quarter cup of flax seed meal. Stir until well mixed. Add 2 spoons of peanut butter and as much cinnamon as you like and keep stirring until you are satisfied with the consistency. Allow a couple of minutes for the mixture to thicken and then enjoy. You can add a few blueberries, either fresh or frozen but no more than a quarter cup.

Lunch: How does chicken meat cooked with vinaigrette accompanied by a chopped romaine or dark green lettuce salad sound? The quantities should be 4 ounces of chicken with 4 cups of the salad.

Snack: Half a cup of almonds

Dinner: Still thinking that you cannot eat steaks? Think again. The day's menu serves pan-fried or grilled steak accompanied by green beans, mushroom and peppers. It's 5 ounces of steak accompanied by a cup of each of the rest.

Menu Suggestion 2:

Breakfast: 3 eggs with a cup of sliced raw mushrooms and half a cup of spinach either scrambled or in omelet, with some cantaloupe on the side (no more than a small slice).

Lunch: Today it's actually a two salad special. One will consist of 6 ounces of tuna, a quarter of a cup walnuts and one large stalk of celery finely chopped, seasoned with cinnamon, salt and pepper to taste. The other will be 3 cups worth of lettuce or romaine salad.

Snack: A nice cup of tea with a single apple flax muffin.

Dinner: Prepare a nice serving of lasagna with shredded mozzarella, parmesan and ricotta cheese and a sauce for spaghetti that is certified sugar free. Accompany with a green salad.

Menu Suggestion 3:

Breakfast: A cup of strained yogurt mixed with half a cup of raspberries and three spoons of sliced almonds.

Lunch: How does a turkey sandwich with asparagus sound? Remember to use low carb bread and no more than three ounces of turkey. The filling should consist from a leaf of lettuce, alfalfa sprouts and mayo. The side dish should contain 8 spears of asparagus.

Snack: A celery stalk with 2 spoons of peanut butter.

Dinner: A pound of chicken breast with beans, a cup of green salad and a dressing as long as it is low carb.

MENU SUGGESTION 4:

Breakfast: All bran cereal with milk (worth half a cup each), 3 spoons of almonds and three quarters of a cup of strawberries.

Lunch: Some bean soup accompanied by two roast beef wraps, lettuce leaves and half a cup of roasted red peppers.

Snack: 15 almonds

Dinner: A very simple dish of unstuffed cabbage.

MENU SUGGESTION 5:

Breakfast: Time for some burritos. You'll need a tortilla, an ounce of ham and 2 scrambled eggs to make the burrito. Serve with 1/8 wedge of cantaloupe.

Lunch: 3 hard-boiled eggs and a large salad of chopped romaine, some raw mushrooms, chopped broccoli and 2 spoons of blue cheese.

Snack: Since it's cheese day, today's snack consists of an ounce of string cheese.

Dinner: About two pounds worth of beef steak with beans, green salad with just one spoon of oil and vinegar dressing and guacamole on the side.

We tried to present a set of suggestions that includes everything. The import thing to remember is to choose foods with low content of carbohydrates. The next chapter will contain the values of the fruits and vegetables that are best suited for this kind of diet and that you can choose from.

FRUIT AND VEGETABLE VALUES IN A KETOGENIC DIET

It is well known that fruits and vegetables are considered as a most essential part of every diet as they contain a multitude of nutrients, anti-inflammatories and anti-oxidants that are of immense value to the human body. However this is not enough for the needs of a ketogenic diet. Their content of effective carbohydrates should also be low enough. Here is a table of the values involved:

Vegetable	Calories	Fiber Content	Effective Carbs
Alfalfa sprouts	8	0.6 grams	0.1 grams
Artichokes	45	7 grams	3 grams
Asparagus	13	1.5 grams	1 gram
Avocado	120	5 grams	1 gram
Bok choy	9	1 gram	1 gram
Broccoli	15	1 gram	2 grams
Brussels sprouts	19	1.5 grams	2 grams
Cabbage	11	1 gram	1.5 grams
Carrots	26	2 grams	4 grams
Cauliflower	12	1 gram	1 gram
Celery	8	1 gram	1 gram
Collards	11	1 gram	1 gram

Cucumbers	45	2 grams	2 grams
Eggplant	17	1 gram	1 gram
Fennel	14	1.5 grams	2 grams
Green beans	17	2 grams	2 grams
Green onions	16	1.5 grams	3 grams
Green peppers	15	1 gram	2,5 grams
Jalapeno peppers	7	0.5 grams	1 gram
Jicama	11	1 gram	1 gram
Leeks	28	1 gram	6.5 grams
Lettuce	3	0.3 grams	0.3 grams
Mung bean sprouts	31	2 grams	4 grams
Mushrooms	8		1 gram
Okra	15	2 grams	2 grams
Onions	32	1 gram	6 grams
Peas	21	1 gram	2,5 grams
Pinto bean sprouts	64	1.5 grams	10 grams
Pumpkin	15	0.5 grams	3.5 grams
Radishes	9	1 gram	1 gram
Red peppers	23	1.5 grams	3 grams
Rutabagas	25	2 grams	4 grams
Spaghetti Squash	21	1 gram	4 grams
Spinach	7	0.7 grams	0.4 grams
Summer squash	12	0.5 grams	1.5 grams
Tomatillos	21	1 gram	3 grams
Tomatoes	16	1 gram	2.5 grams

Turnips	18	1 gram	3 grams
Zucchini	10	1 gram	1.5 grams

All the values mentioned in the above list refer to each vegetable when it is consumed raw and uncooked. If one was to search online they would find plenty of references to the respective values for cooked or boiled forms of the same vegetables.

Water chestnuts, beets, butternut, acorn and parsnips have too high of an effective carbohydrate content to be included in a ketogenic diet and should be avoided. Furthermore, it is strongly recommended that organically grown vegetables are preferred over regularly grown ones as less chemicals have been involved in their cultivation.

The second part that refers to fruits is a little bit more complicated. There is a number of scientists who maintain that originally humans were designed to be fruit eaters instead of carnivores or even vegetable consumers.

The complication comes from a strong debate within the scientific community about the need to include fruits in a ketogenic diet. A contingent of scientists maintains that the sugar content should not be calculated in the values of each fruit and that only their carbohydrate content should be taken into account.

Another contingent thinks that the glycemic load is of higher importance and should not be excluded when fruits are considered as suggestions in a menu. The following list contains both values used by most professionals when they make their suggestions:

Fruit form	Glycemic load	Effective Carbs	Calories
1 medium peach	5	12 grams	59
1 medium stalk	1	2 grams	11
1 wedge of casaba melon	4	10 grams	46
1 wedge of watermelon	6	22 grams	86
Blackberries	2	3.5 grams	31
Casaba melon cubs	2	1 gram	24
Chopped apple	4	7 grams	32
Chopped cranberries	1	4 grams	25
Cranberries	0	2 grams	13
Cubed cantaloupe	2	7 grams	26
Diced Rhubarb	1	1.5 grams	13
Diced watermelon	1.5	5.5 grams	23
Fresh blueberries	3	9 grams	42
Fresh lemon juice	1	1 gram	4
Fresh lime juice	0	1 gram	11
Fresh raspberries	1.5	3.5 grams	32
Frozen blackberries	2	8 grams	49
Frozen blueberries	3	7 grams	40
Frozen raspberries	1.5	6 grams	32
Juice of 1 medium lemon	1	4 grams	12
Juice of 1 medium lime	1	4 grams	11
Large strawberry	0	1 gram	6

Med wedge cantaloupe	2	6 grams	23
Medium apple	6	21 grams	95
Medium nectarine	5	13 grams	62
Medium papaya	7	25 grams	119
Papaya cubes	1.5	6 grams	27
Sliced nectarines	2.5	6 grams	31
Sliced peaches	3	6.5 grams	30
Sliced strawberries	1.5	5 grams	26

One thing to always remember is that fruits are good if consumed in certain quantities only. Otherwise they fall outside the limits set by a ketogenic diet and they will cause the production of glucose which will offset the designing of the diet.

The next step in our journey into a ketogenic diet will dig a little deeper into some very serious concepts that most of us tend to ignore at our own risk.

BREAKFAST: THE MOST IMPORTANT MEAL OF THE DAY

One of the greatest mistakes we all do is to get up in the morning and have nothing more than a cup of coffee (if we have one at all) before we rush out to get to work. Every doctor in every discipline will tell you that this is a fundamental error as it is breakfast that is the meal that will replenish the energy supplies that you need for the coming day. Energy is the basic concept of the ketogenic diet.

Let's discuss what must be included in a daily breakfast so that the diet is not disrupted:

CEREALS

On this category we can all agree that they are both tasty and do not take too long to prepare. This latest issue is most crucial as time is always pressing. Children love it and adults have always favored it. To include them in a ketogenic diet you must look either for the low carb varieties that are available in the market, or for the ones that are rich in fiber content.

EGGS

Is there anyone who is not fond of a scrambled eggs, bacon and jam breakfast? We know we all love it but the greatest issue again is the time it takes to prepare it.

However, if you are in a ketogenic diet you must forget all the rest and keep only the eggs out of such a breakfast.

Eggs are among the most precious foods you are up to find and there are thousands of fast recipes you can use. If necessary prepare your breakfast the night before and do not avoid eating it in the morning. There is no restriction on the form to prepare other than the number of eggs to consume which will be determined by your attending physician.

DAIRY PRODUCTS

Cottage cheese, yogurt, tofu and ricotta are ideal for a ketogenic diet. For better results mix them with fruit or a protein powder.

BREADS

The idea of slices with butter and jam is to be forgotten (unfortunately but necessary). If you want any kind of bread with your breakfast you will need to bake it yourself choosing ingredients that have low effective carbs.

There is another reason that you need to consider the need for breakfast. Having just a cup of coffee will actually negate your entire effort to change your body to using ketones instead of glucose. Coffee may be a stimulant and help you wake up, but it does not provide the body with any usable energy through glucose or through the production of ketones. What it will do, is take your body out of ketosis and all your efforts will have been in vain.

Therefore you will definitely need to consider either waking up a little earlier in the morning to have ample time to prepare your breakfast or have someone else prepare it for you, or make arrangements for a previous night preparation.

The last remaining issue to discuss is the need for snacks. In the modern world this is probably one of the greatest mistakes we do and it will destroy all our efforts to remain fit if specific issues are not taken into account. This is what the next chapter is for.

Who says you can't eat snacks?

It is an unfortunate reality but if you turn into a ketogenic diet after years of being used to eating snacks all day long it will be extremely hard for you to get rid of this habit. We all know that an axiom in life is that there is no stronger force than the power of habit.

However, you do not need to worry that a ketogenic diet will take this habit completely out of your life. But you will need to adjust to a new set of snacks and to eat them only when you feel low on energy and hungry between meals. There is an entire list to select from:

✓ ¼ cup of berries with 1/3 cup of cottage cheese

✓ 4 ounces yogurt (plain)

✓ Cheddar cheese with dill pickles

✓ Cheese sticks

✓ Cheese with some slices of apple

✓ Cucumber slices with cream cheese and smoked salmon

✓ Deviled eggs

✓ Garlic crackers with parmesan

✓ Hard boiled eggs

✓ Jell-o that is sugar free with cottage cheese and nuts

- ✓ Lettuce roll-ups (with luncheon meat, egg salad, tuna, or any other filling)
- ✓ Low sugar varieties of jerky (either beef or turkey)
- ✓ Mushrooms with cheese spread
- ✓ Nuts
- ✓ Peanut butter with celery
- ✓ Pepperoni "chips" (pepperoni slices in the microwave oven)
- ✓ Pork rinds
- ✓ Raw vegetables with spinach dip
- ✓ Ricotta cheese with fruit.
- ✓ Snack bars as long as they are low-carb without sugar alcohols and without maltitol.
- ✓ Tuna salad with celery

All the above combinations and suggestions are low in effective carbs and just with the right amounts of fat so that your body remains in ketosis. There is even some fiber and some protein included so that the balance is not upset.

There are millions of combinations that you can search for online. Just remember to include their value into your everyday calculations of the effective carbohydrates, protein and fat consumed. The balance is crucial but does allow for some latitude which you are not to exceed otherwise your body will be taken out of ketosis.

There is no doubt that a ketogenic diet is a rather hard diet to follow and one that requires constant supervision and changes. But as the saying goes there is nothing that is worth doing that is easy. It's just a matter of decision. And you need to make that decision.

Conclusion:

The entire idea behind a ketogenic diet is to force the body to adjust to a new set of habits. Glucose is the easy way to energy with the side effect that the weight control may be easily lost resulting in a constant need for reducing the amount of food consumed or going through vigorous physical activity to maintain the proper weight.

Switching from glucose to ketones may save you this kind of trouble. As before mentioned, people that follow this diet are compelled not to eat too much anyway. However, there is something of even more importance than the body that has to be adjusted and that is your own mind.

Every diet must include a very significant mental component. Either that being the need to lose the extra weight, or the necessity to follow the instructions of your attending physician in order to remedy a medical condition, it is not enough. You need to think and convince yourself that this is the best course of action for you.

If you need to consider the bonuses of a ketogenic diet, think that it is not as restricting to what you can eat for other diets. You can sort through the available options and combinations until you find a weekly set that will be to your absolute liking.

Furthermore, if you do not like ready-made foods, you can indulge in the myriads of recipes that are available online and are open to experimentation as long as you do not exceed the limitations set by your own goals. If you do experiment it is strongly recommended that you test your creations first to see if they fit into the profile set by the physician that has designed your program.

We have repeatedly mentioned the need for a supervising professional. Let's add two more reasons to this need. The first one being that they are the only ones qualified to detect whether there is a problem arising that should force the termination of the program and the selection of another one.

The second one is to help you re-adjust to a glucose based diet should your body be unable to adjust to the production of ketones or to remain in nutritional ketosis. This is the last part that you should really be aware of.

If your body manages to adjust to nutritional ketosis, abandoning this diet will be extremely difficult not to mention thoroughly unpleasant. This is why we tell you to think long and hard about the benefits of this diet. Once you get into it you will get into it for good. Isn't this more worth doing than following hundreds of different diets and all they do is bring temporary results if any at all?

In fact if the hardship to be suffered in a diet is any indication, then a ketogenic diet is by far a similar concept to becoming a champion of a sport. So you need to consider whether you want to be a champion or just another one who spends fortunes on nutritionists for doubtful results.

www.ingramcontent.com/pod-product-compliance
Lightning Source LLC
Chambersburg PA
CBHW070245290526
45789CB00004B/1766